Health Information Management - Health Information Service, Clinical Coding, Governance, and Digital Transformation in Modern Healthcare

HTET MYAT AUNG ZAW

Published by HTET MYAT AUNG ZAW, 2026.

HEALTH INFORMATION MANAGEMENT - HEALTH INFORMATION SERVICE, CLINICAL CODING, GOVERNANCE, AND DIGITAL TRANSFORMATION IN MODERN HEALTHCARE

First edition. August 31, 2026.

ISBN: 979-8235839946

Written by HTET MYAT AUNG ZAW.

FOREWORD

Written by Htet Myat Aung Zaw, Senior Health Information Manager

Health Information Management is one of the most strategically important disciplines in modern healthcare. At its core lies a profession that safeguards patient information, strengthens digital transformation, and ensures the financial sustainability of hospitals through accurate, ethical, and high-quality data.

Among the most critical contributors to this mission are Health Information Managers and Clinical Coders. Their work includes interpreting clinical documentation and assigning accurate ICD-10-AM and ACHI codes, directly determining the Diagnosis Related Group (DRG) assigned to each patient episode. These DRGs form the foundation of Activity-Based Funding (ABF), influencing millions of dollars in casemix-based revenue every year. Coding accuracy is not simply a technical task; it is a financial, clinical, and governance responsibility that shapes hospital performance, resource allocation, and patient outcomes.

Throughout my career, I have seen how powerful Health Information Management (HIM) can be when Health Information Managers, Clinical Coders, Analysts, Privacy Officers, FOI Officers, and Digital Health Leaders work together. HIM professionals are the custodians of information integrity, ensuring that documentation reflects true clinical care, that coding is precise and compliant, and that funding is fair, transparent, and defensible.

This book brings together the essential elements of HIM practice, highlighting the importance of coding, documentation quality, governance, digital health, leadership, and future-focused capability. It is written for professionals and students who carry the responsibility of managing information that influences clinical safety, organisational reputation, and multimillion-dollar funding outcomes.

I am honoured to present this work to the HIM community. May it strengthen your confidence, deepen your expertise, and inspire the next generation of HIM leaders and Clinical Coders.

Htet Myat Aung Zaw
Senior Health Information Manager
Melbourne, Australia

PREFACE

Clinical coding is one of the most vital components of Health Information Management. HIMs and Clinical Coders transform complex clinical documentation into structured data that drives Activity-Based Funding (ABF), national reporting, research, and performance monitoring. Every diagnosis, procedure, comorbidity, and complication must be coded with precision, as even a single missed condition can alter a DRG and impact thousands or millions of dollars in hospital revenue.

This book recognises the essential role of HIMs and Clinical Coders, and HIM professionals in managing casemix complexity and funding integrity. HIM teams ensure that documentation is complete, coding is accurate, audits are robust, and data reflects the true clinical picture. They are responsible for safeguarding the financial sustainability of hospitals, supporting clinicians, and upholding ethical governance.

The chapters in this book provide a comprehensive overview of HIM practice, including digital health, privacy, FOI, data quality, leadership, and future-focused career development. They are written to support both new and experienced professionals who contribute to the financial, clinical, and ethical foundations of healthcare.

My hope is that this book strengthens professional identity, supports lifelong learning, and highlights the profound impact HIM professionals especially Health Information Managers and Clinical Coders have on the health systems.

BOOK INTRODUCTION

Health Information Management (HIM) is one of the most essential and strategic disciplines in modern healthcare. At the heart of this profession are Health Information Managers (HIMs) who are leaders overseeing the entire lifecycle of health information, from documentation and coding to privacy, FOI, digital health, analytics, and governance. HIMs ensure that information is accurate, secure, ethical, and used responsibly to support patient care, organisational performance, and financial sustainability.

HIMs lead multidisciplinary teams that include Clinical Coders, Privacy Officers, FOI Officers, Digital Health Specialists, Casemix Managers, Coding Auditors, and Information Governance Managers. Together, they safeguard patient rights, uphold legislative compliance, strengthen digital transformation, and manage multimillion-dollar casemix portfolios that determine hospital funding under Activity-Based Funding (ABF).

This book provides a comprehensive, future-focused exploration of HIM practice across six core domains: foundational principles, digital health, data quality and funding integrity, privacy and FOI, leadership and workforce development, and long-term career growth. It is written for Health Information Managers, Clinical Coders, and all professionals who contribute to the safe, ethical, and high-performing management of health information.

Readers will gain a deep understanding of how HIMs:

- Lead Clinical Coders and oversee coding accuracy, DRG assignment, and casemix integrity
- Protect patient rights through privacy, confidentiality, and ethical information release
- Strengthen digital health transformation through EMR optimisation, interoperability, automation, and cybersecurity
- Ensure data quality and reporting accuracy through

documentation improvement, coding excellence, and robust auditing
- Manage multimillion-dollar casemix portfolios and safeguard ABF funding integrity
- Lead teams, influence stakeholders, and build psychologically safe workplaces
- Develop professional identity, digital resilience, and global competence
- Prepare for emerging roles in AI, interoperability, digital governance, and advanced analytics

While Clinical Coders play a vital role in transforming documentation into coded data, HIMs provide the leadership, governance, and strategic oversight that ensures this information is accurate, compliant, and financially defensible. HIMs are the stewards of information integrity and the architects of digital health transformation.

With practical insights, professional frameworks, and future-focused strategies, this book serves as a complete guide for anyone seeking to thrive in the evolving HIM landscape. Whether you are beginning your career or advancing into leadership, this text provides the knowledge, confidence, and inspiration needed to contribute meaningfully to safe, ethical, and high-performing healthcare systems.

About the Author

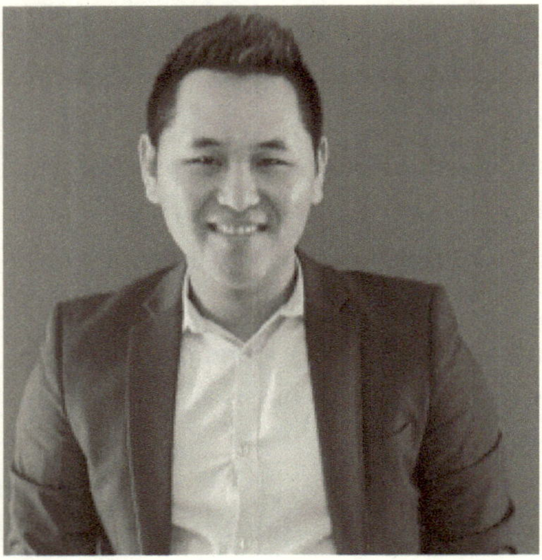

Htet Myat Aung Zaw is an accomplished Health Information Manager (Clinical Coder) with extensive experience across public and private healthcare organisations in Australia. He has served in multiple leadership roles, including Chief Health Information Manager (Acting) and Manager of Health Information Management and Client Applications, where he has led teams in clinical coding, privacy compliance, Freedom of Information (FOI), digital health transformation, and information governance.

Htet Myat Aung holds a Master of Health Information Management from La Trobe University, a Bachelor of Biomedical Science from Deakin University, and completed a Master of Arts in Christian Studies at Hillsong College affiliated with Alphacrucis University College, reflecting his commitment to ethical leadership, compassion, and integrity in healthcare.

In addition to his professional work, Htet Myat Aung is an Australian Christian Churches accredited Pastor, serving the community at Victory International Church in the Western Melbourne region. His pastoral ministry strengthens his dedication to supporting individuals, families, and communities with care, guidance, and faith-based leadership.

Throughout his career, Htet Myat Aung has championed excellence in clinical coding, data quality, digital health innovation, and information governance, empowering Health Information Managers and Clinical Coders to lead with professionalism, accuracy, and humanity.

Chapter 1: Foundations of Health Information Management

Introduction

Health Information Management (HIM) is the backbone of modern healthcare systems. HIM is a strategic discipline that underpins safe, ethical, and high-performing healthcare systems. At the centre of this profession are Health Information Managers (HIMs) who are leaders overseeing the creation, protection, analysis, and governance of health information. HIMs ensure that information is accurate, secure, and used responsibly to support patient care, organisational performance, and legislative compliance.

HIMs lead multidisciplinary teams including Clinical Coders, Privacy Officers, FOI Officers, Digital Health Specialists, Casemix Managers, and Information Governance Managers. Together, they safeguard patient rights, uphold ethical standards, and ensure the integrity of health information across its entire lifecycle.

The Role and Scope of Health Information Managers (HIMs)

HIMs intersects with multidisciplinary profession including clinical documentation, privacy, digital health, governance, analytics, and organisational strategy. HIMs professionals ensure that information supports safe, ethical, and efficient healthcare delivery.

HIMs are responsible for:

- Managing Clinical Coders and coding operations
- Overseeing privacy, FOI, and information release
- Leading clinical documentation and coding
- Leading digital health transformation
- Ensuring documentation and data quality
- Managing casemix and ABF funding integrity
- Implementing governance frameworks
- Educating clinicians and executives

- Leading audits and compliance activities
- Supporting medico-legal and risk management processes
- Records management
- Health analytics
- Cybersecurity

IFHIMA (2022) describes HIM professionals as "guardians of health information integrity," highlighting the profession's global significance. HIMs are also both operational leaders and strategic advisors.

Core Principles of HIM Practice

HIM practice is grounded in several foundational principles:

Accuracy

Information must reflect the true clinical scenario.

Confidentiality

Patient information must be protected from unauthorised access.

Integrity

Data must be complete, consistent, and trustworthy.

Accessibility

Information must be available to authorised users when needed.

Accountability

HIM professionals must uphold ethical and legislative standards.

These principles underpin all HIM functions, from coding to privacy to digital health.

Privacy and Confidentiality in Healthcare

Privacy is a fundamental human right and a core HIM responsibility. Key legislation includes:

- *Privacy Act 1988*
- Australian Privacy Principles (APPs)

- *Health Records Act 2001* (Vic)
- *Health Records and Information Privacy Act 2002* (NSW)
- GDPR (Europe)
- HIPAA (United States)

The Office of the Australian Information Commissioner (OAIC, 2024) emphasises that privacy compliance protects patient rights and strengthens public trust.

Key Privacy Obligations

- Collect only necessary information
- Use information for legitimate purposes
- Secure data against breaches
- Provide access to individuals upon request
- Maintain transparency about information handling

Privacy breaches can result in legal penalties, reputational damage, and patient harm.

Freedom of Information (FOI) in Healthcare

FOI legislation promotes transparency and accountability by allowing individuals to request access to documents held by public agencies.

FOI Principles

- Right of access
- Timely response
- Clear reasoning
- Fairness and impartiality
- Protection of sensitive information

FOI Workflow

FOI decision-making involves:

- Receiving and validating requests
- Locating relevant documents
- Assessing exemptions
- Consulting with stakeholders
- Applying the public interest test
- Issuing written decisions
- Releasing documents or refusing access

OVIC (2021) emphasises that FOI decision-making requires strong legislative knowledge and ethical judgment.

Common FOI Exemptions

- Personal privacy
- Legal professional privilege
- Health and safety risks
- Law enforcement
- Cabinet documents
- Confidential commercial information

FOI is a high-stakes HIM function requiring accuracy, fairness, and transparency.

Information Governance in Healthcare

Information governance ensures that health information is managed ethically, securely, and in compliance with legislation.

Key Components

- Privacy
- FOI
- Records management
- Cybersecurity
- Data quality
- Risk management
- Policy development

- Compliance monitoring

The Australian Digital Health Agency (ADHA, 2024) emphasises that governance is essential for safe digital health environments.

Records Management

Governed by:

- *Public Records Act 1973* (Vic)
- State archival authorities
- National digital health standards

Records must be accurate, complete, secure, retained appropriately, and disposed of lawfully.

Global Perspectives on HIM

HIM is expanding globally due to digital health adoption, privacy regulation, and interoperability initiatives.

Global Trends

- ICD-11 adoption
- SNOMED CT expansion
- AI-assisted coding
- Telehealth growth
- Cloud-based EMRs
- International data sharing
- Global privacy frameworks

WHO (2023) emphasises that global digital health maturity is essential for safe and equitable healthcare.

Pathways to Becoming a Health Information Manager

Becoming a **Health Information Manager (HIM)** typically requires formal tertiary education in Health Information Management or a closely related discipline. In Australia, HIMs are usually qualified through:

- **Bachelor of Health Information Management** (3 years)
- **Master of Health Information Management** (2 years postgraduate)
- **Equivalent international HIM degrees** recognised by IFHIMA
- **Additional certifications** in privacy, FOI, digital health, or data governance (optional but advantageous)

HIMs often come from backgrounds in:

- Medicine
- Biomedical science
- Nursing
- IT and digital health
- Health administration
- Data science
- Allied Health

Professional membership with **HIMAA** or **IFHIMA** is strongly encouraged for career development, continuing education, and professional recognition.

Salary Expectations for Foundational HIM Roles

Australia (2024–2026)

Sources: Seek, Indeed, Labour Market Insights.

- HIM Officer: AUD $70,000–$85,000
- FOI/Privacy Officer: AUD $80,000–$105,000
- Clinical Coder: AUD $65,000–$80,000
- Records Officer: AUD $60,000–$75,000

- Senior HIM Officer: AUD $95,000–$120,000
- Team Leader / Supervisor: AUD $100,000–$130,000
- HIM Manager: AUD $120,000–$150,000

- Information Governance Manager: AUD $120,000–$150,000
- Director of Health Information Services: AUD $160,000–$220,000

United States (AHIMA, 2024)

- HIM Technician: USD $45,000–$60,000
- Privacy Analyst: USD $70,000–$95,000
- HIM Manager: USD $80,000–$120,000
- Director of HIM: USD $120,000–$160,000
- Chief Health Information Officer: USD $180,000–$250,000

United Kingdom (NHS, 2024)

- Information Officer: £28,000–£35,000
- FOI Officer: £30,000–£38,000

- Senior Information Manager: £45,000–£55,000
- Head of Information Governance: £50,000–£65,000
- Director of Digital Health: £75,000–£130,000

Learning Framework: Building Strong HIM Foundations

- Study legislation — Privacy, FOI, records management
- Develop digital literacy — EMRs, cybersecurity basics
- Strengthen communication skills — Clear, respectful, professional
- Practice ethical decision-making — Fairness, transparency, integrity
- Engage in professional development — HIMAA, AHIMA, IFHIMA
- Build foundational technical skills — Coding, documentation, data quality

Conclusion

Foundational HIM practice is essential for safe, ethical, and efficient healthcare. Privacy, FOI, governance, and digital literacy form the core of the profession. As healthcare evolves, HIM professionals must uphold integrity, accuracy, and accountability while adapting to new technologies and global standards.

Chapter 2: Digital Health, Systems, and Interoperability

Digital health is transforming healthcare systems worldwide. Electronic medical records, artificial intelligence, automation, interoperability standards, and cybersecurity frameworks are reshaping how information is captured, stored, shared, and used. Health Information Management (HIM) professionals play a central role in guiding organisations through this transformation, ensuring that digital systems support safe, efficient, and ethical healthcare delivery.

This chapter explores digital health foundations, interoperability, AI-assisted coding, automation, cybersecurity, and global digital health trends.

Digital Health in Modern Healthcare

Digital health refers to the use of digital technologies to improve health outcomes, enhance system performance, and strengthen patient experience. The Australian Digital Health Agency (ADHA, 2024) defines digital health as the strategic integration of digital tools across clinical, administrative, and governance domains.

Key digital health components include:

- Electronic medical records (EMRs)
- Electronic health records (EHRs)
- Patient Administrative systems (PAS)
- Clinical information systems (CIS)
- Digital identity systems
- Telehealth platforms
- Consumer health apps
- Cloud-based data storage
- Cybersecurity frameworks

Digital health maturity is now a core indicator of healthcare quality and safety.

Electronic Medical Records and System Integration

EMRs and EHRs are central to digital health. They support:

- Clinical Documentation
- Medication Management
- Diagnostic Results
- Care Coordination
- Patient Engagement
- Reporting And Analytics
- Health Information Management Services
- Clinical Coding
- Freedom Of Information & Release Of Information

HIM professionals ensure that EMR data is accurate, complete, and compliant with privacy legislation.

Key EMR Responsibilities for HIM Professionals

- Documentation quality audits
- Data validation
- Workflow optimisation
- Privacy and access controls
- System configuration input
- Training and support for clinical staff

Effective EMR use improves patient safety, reduces duplication, and enhances clinical decision-making.

Interoperability and Standards

Interoperability enables seamless data exchange across systems, organisations, and jurisdictions. It is essential for continuity of care, national reporting, and digital health maturity.

Core Interoperability Standards

- **HL7** — messaging standard for clinical data exchange
- **ICD-10-AM / ICD-11** — classification systems for morbidity and mortality
- **FHIR** — modern API-based standard enabling real-time data sharing
- **SNOMED CT** — global clinical terminology
- **LOINC** — laboratory and clinical observation codes

ADHA (2024) emphasises that interoperability is a national priority for Australia's digital health future.

Benefits of Interoperability

- Reduced duplication
- Improved patient safety
- Faster access to information
- Enhanced analytics
- Better coordination across care settings
- Stronger national reporting
- Accurate, effective and efficient coding

Interoperability is a critical HIM competency in modern healthcare.

Artificial Intelligence in Health Information Management

Artificial intelligence (AI) is reshaping HIM practice, particularly in clinical coding, documentation improvement, and data quality.

AI-Assisted Coding

AI tools use natural language processing (NLP) to interpret clinical documentation and suggest codes.

Benefits include:

- Faster coding turnaround
- Improved accuracy for common diagnoses
- Real-time documentation feedback
- Enhanced audit trails

AHIMA (2024) emphasises that AI supports but does not replace human Clinical Coders. HIM professionals must validate AI outputs, apply coding standards, and ensure compliance.

AI in Data Quality

Machine learning models detect:

- Missing data
- Logical inconsistencies
- Documentation gaps
- Anomalies in reporting

AI strengthens data integrity and supports funding accuracy.

Automation and Workflow Optimisation

Automation improves efficiency and reduces manual workload across HIM functions.

Common Automation Tools

- Robotic Process Automation (RPA)
- Automated FOI redaction tools
- Auto-routing of requests and tasks
- Digital forms and workflows
- Automated data validation scripts

IFHIMA (2022) notes that automation reduces human error and supports consistent data quality.

Automation Benefits

- Faster turnaround times
- Reduced administrative burden
- Improved accuracy
- Enhanced compliance
- Better staff satisfaction

Automation is essential for modern HIM practice.

Cybersecurity and Digital Risk Management

Digital transformation increases cybersecurity risks. HIM professionals must understand cybersecurity principles to protect patient information.

Common Cybersecurity Threats

- Ransomware
- Data breaches
- Identity theft
- Insider threats
- Cloud vulnerabilities

Key Cybersecurity Controls

- Access management
- Encryption
- Multi-factor authentication
- Audit logs
- Incident response plans
- Regular risk assessments

The Office of the Australian Information Commissioner (OAIC, 2024) emphasises that cybersecurity is both a legal and ethical obligation.

Cybersecurity literacy is now a core HIM competency.

Global Digital Health Trends

Digital health is expanding worldwide, driven by technological innovation, consumer expectations, and global health priorities.

Major Global Trends

- Adoption of ICD-11
- Expansion of SNOMED CT

- Growth of telehealth and virtual care
- AI-driven clinical decision support
- Cloud-based EMRs
- Digital identity and patient portals
- International data sharing
- Global privacy frameworks (GDPR, HIPAA)

WHO (2023) emphasises that global digital health maturity is essential for safe, equitable healthcare.

HIM professionals must understand global trends to remain competitive and future-ready.

Qualifications for Digital Health Specialists

Digital Health Specialists typically hold qualifications in:

- **Health Information Management**
- **Information Technology**
- **Computer Science**
- **Health Informatics**
- **Cybersecurity**
- **Data Science**

Additional certifications include:

- **HIMSS Digital Health Certifications**
- **Cybersecurity certifications** (CompTIA Security+, CISSP)
- **Vendor-specific EMR training** (Cerner, Epic, Meditech)
- **Interoperability training** (HL7, FHIR, SNOMED CT)

HIMs often progress into digital health leadership roles due to their strong understanding of clinical workflows, data standards, and governance.

Salary Expectations for Digital Health and Interoperability Roles

Australia (2024–2026)

Sources: Seek, Indeed, Labour Market Insights.

- Digital Health Officer: AUD $95,000–$125,000
- Systems Analyst (Health): AUD $100,000–$135,000
- Interoperability Specialist: AUD $115,000–$145,000
- AI-Assisted Coding Specialist: AUD $105,000–$140,000
- Digital Health Manager: AUD $130,000–$160,000

United States (HIMSS, 2024)

- Health IT Specialist: USD $75,000–$105,000
- Clinical Systems Analyst: USD $90,000–$125,000
- Chief Health Information Officer: USD $180,000–$250,000

United Kingdom (NHS, 2024)

- Digital Systems Manager: £45,000–£55,000
- Health Informatics Specialist: £32,000–£42,000
- Head of Digital Health: £55,000–£75,000

Learning Framework: Strengthening Digital Health Capability

- Develop EMR/EHR literacy
- Master interoperability standards
- Learn AI and automation tools
- Strengthen cybersecurity awareness
- Participate in digital health projects
- Engage with HIMSS, AHIMA, IFHIMA
- Pursue digital health certifications
- Build analytical and technical skills

Conclusion

Digital health is transforming the HIM profession. Interoperability, AI, automation, and cybersecurity are now essential competencies for HIM professionals. By embracing digital innovation and strengthening technical capability, HIM professionals can lead safe, efficient, and future-ready healthcare systems.

Chapter 3: Data Quality, Clinical Coding, Reporting, and Funding Integrity

High-quality health data is the foundation of safe patient care, accurate reporting, transparent governance, and sustainable hospital funding. Health Information Management (HIM) professionals particularly Health Information Managers, Clinical Coders, Data Analysts, and Documentation Specialists play a critical role in ensuring that clinical information is complete, accurate, and compliant with national standards.

The Australian Institute of Health and Welfare (AIHW, 2024) emphasises that data quality is essential for health system performance, influencing everything from Activity-Based Funding (ABF) to national reporting, clinical benchmarking, and strategic decision-making. This chapter explores clinical documentation, coding accuracy, casemix complexity, ABF, national reporting, analytics, and the financial stewardship HIM professionals provide.

The Importance of Data Quality in Healthcare

Data quality determines the reliability of clinical, administrative, and financial information. Poor-quality data can lead to:

- Incorrect funding
- Misleading performance indicators
- Compromised patient safety
- Inaccurate national reporting
- Ineffective clinical decision-making
- Increased organisational risk

High-quality data supports transparency, accountability, and evidence-based care.

Key Dimensions of Data Quality

- **Accuracy** — data reflects the true clinical scenario
- **Completeness** — all required fields are present
- **Consistency** — data aligns across systems
- **Timeliness** — data is available when needed
- **Validity** — data meets format and logic rules
- **Reliability** — data is dependable over time

HIM professionals ensure these dimensions through audits, validation, documentation improvement, and coding quality initiatives.

Clinical Documentation: The Foundation of Accurate Coding

Clinical documentation is the primary source of truth for coding and reporting. High quality documentation ensures:

- Accurate ICD-10-AM and ACHI coding
- Correct DRG assignment
- Reliable ABF funding
- Meaningful clinical communication
- Strong medico-legal protection

Common Documentation Issues

- Missing diagnoses
- Incomplete procedures
- Ambiguous terminology
- Lack of specificity
- Poor linkage between clinical notes and coded data

HIM professionals work closely with clinicians to improve documentation through education, audits, and feedback.

Clinical Coding: Transforming Documentation into Funding and Intelligence

Clinical Coders interpret complex clinical documentation and translate it into structured data using ICD-10-AM, ACHI, and Australian Coding Standards (ACS). Their work directly influences:

- Hospital funding
- Performance indicators
- National reporting
- Research and analytics
- Clinical benchmarking
- Organisational risk management

Coding accuracy is essential for ensuring that hospitals receive fair reimbursement for the care they provide.

The Financial Impact of Coding Accuracy

Under Activity-Based Funding:

- Each coded episode generates a Diagnosis Related Group (DRG)
- Each DRG has a National Weighted Activity Unit (NWAU)
- Each NWAU has a dollar value set by IHACPA
- Incorrect coding can lead to under-funding or over-funding
- Funding discrepancies can reach hundreds of thousands or millions of dollars

Clinical Coders and HIM professionals therefore act as financial stewards, ensuring that hospitals receive accurate, defensible, and transparent funding.

Examples of Coding-Driven Funding Impacts

- Missing a significant comorbidity (e.g., sepsis, acute renal failure) can shift a DRG and reduce funding by thousands of dollars.
- Incorrect procedure coding (e.g., failing to code a major

surgical intervention) can lead to substantial under-funding.
- Over-coding or incorrect sequencing can trigger audits, repayments, and compliance risks.

Accurate coding protects both financial integrity and clinical credibility.

Casemix Complexity and HIM Leadership

Casemix describes the mix of patient care types treated by a hospital. It is used for:

- Funding allocation
- Benchmarking
- Performance analysis
- Resource planning
- Strategic decision-making

HIM professionals manage casemix complexity by:

- Leading coding audits
- Ensuring documentation completeness
- Monitoring DRG shifts
- Identifying comorbidity capture trends
- Collaborating with clinicians and finance teams
- Ensuring compliance with IHACPA standards
- Supporting clinical documentation improvement (CDI) programs

Casemix management is a multimillion-dollar responsibility requiring advanced analytical skills, clinical understanding, and governance expertise.

Activity-Based Funding (ABF): The Financial Engine of Australian Hospitals

ABF is the primary funding model for Australian hospitals. It allocates funding based on the complexity and volume of patient care.

How ABF Works

ABF uses coded data to group episodes into DRGs. Funding is influenced by:

- Principal diagnosis
- Comorbidities
- Procedures
- Length of stay
- Complications
- Patient demographics

IHACPA (2022) emphasises that accurate coding and documentation are essential for fair and transparent funding.

The Role of HIM in ABF Integrity

HIM professionals ensure:

- Accurate DRG assignment
- Correct NWAU calculation
- Reliable cost-weight application
- Transparent audit trails
- Compliance with national standards

ABF integrity is essential for hospital sustainability and public trust.

National and State Reporting Requirements

Hospitals must submit high-quality data to national and state agencies.

National Health Repositories & Functional Frameworks

Regardless of the state or territory, data from across Australia is universally funnelled into these centralized federal repositories managed by the **AIHW** and **IHACPA**:

Activity, Costing & Outpatient Repositories

- **NHMD:** National Hospital Morbidity Database (compiles all state/territory admitted inpatient data)
- **NHCDC:** National Hospital Cost Data Collection (gathers costing data to set the National Efficient Price for funding)
- **NHDH:** National Health Data Hub (consolidates non-admitted and community care activity)

Specialized Disease & Public Health Repositories

- **ACD:** Australian Cancer Database (consolidates all state and territory cancer registries)
- **NPDC:** National Perinatal Data Collection (aggregates nationwide birth and maternal health outcomes)
- **AODTS NMDS:** Alcohol and Other Drug Treatment Services National Minimum Data Set
- **NCMHCD:** National Community Mental Health Care Database

Sub-Acute Care, Mental Health & Aged Care Networks

- **AROC:** Australian Rehabilitation Outcomes Centre (uses the **FIM** — Functional Independence Measure instrument)
- **PCOC:** Palliative Care Outcomes Collaboration
- **PMHC MDS:** Primary Mental Health Care Minimum Data Set (collected via Primary Health Networks)
- **NOCC:** National Outcomes and Casemix Collection (tracks clinical outcomes like HoNOS scales)
- **AN-ACC Framework:** Australian National Aged Care Classification (managed via the **My Aged Care Portal** and **NQI** safety program)
- **AOANJRR:** Australian Orthopaedic Association National Joint Replacement Registry

Key Reporting Datasets from different states include:
Victoria (VIC)

- **Admitted Inpatients: VAED** (Victorian Admitted Episodes Dataset)
- **Emergency Department: VEMD** (Victorian Emergency Minimum Dataset)
- **Outpatients & Community: VAPC** (Victorian Ambulatory Plasma Collection), **VINAH** (Victorian Integrated Non-Admitted Health)
- **Mental Health: CMI/ODS** (Client Management Interface / Operational Data Store)
- **Alcohol and Other Drugs: VADC** (Victorian Alcohol and Drug Collection)
- **Statutory Registries: VCR** (Victorian Cancer Registry), **VPDC** (Victorian Perinatal Data Collection)
- **Clinical Quality & Trauma: VSTR** (Victorian State Trauma Registry), **VCOR** (Victorian Cardiac Outcomes Registry)

New South Wales (NSW)

- **Admitted Inpatients: APDC** (Admitted Patient Data Collection)
- **Emergency Department: EDDC** (Emergency Department Data Collection)
- **Outpatients / Ambulatory: NAPDC** (Non-Admitted Patient Data Collection)
- **Statutory Registries: NSWCR** (New South Wales Cancer Registry), **NSWPDC** (NSW Perinatal Data Collection)

Queensland (QLD)

- **Admitted Inpatients: QHAPDC** (Queensland Hospital Admitted Patient Data Collection)
- **Emergency Department: EDIS / EDDC** (Emergency Department Information System / Data Collection)
- **Statutory Registries: QCR** (Queensland Cancer Registry), **QPDC** (Queensland Perinatal Data Collection)

Western Australia (WA)

- **Admitted Inpatients: HMDS** (Hospital Morbidity Data System)
- **Emergency Department: EDDC** (Emergency Department Data Collection)
- **Statutory Registries: WACR** (Western Australian Cancer Registry), **WAPDC** (Western Australian Perinatal Data Collection)

South Australia (SA)

- **Admitted Inpatients: APC** (Admitted Patient Care), historically known as **ISAAC** (Integrated South Australian Activity Collection)
- **Emergency Department: ED Presentations Dataset**
- **Statutory Registries: SACR** (South Australian Cancer Registry), **SAPDC** (South Australian Perinatal Data Collection)

Tasmania (TAS)

- **Admitted Inpatients: TAPDS** (Tasmanian Admitted Patient Data Set)
- **Emergency Department: TEDD** (Tasmanian Emergency

Department Dataset)

- **Statutory Registries: TCR** (Tasmanian Cancer Registry), **TPDC** (Tasmanian Perinatal Data Collection)

Australian Capital Territory (ACT)

- **Admitted Inpatients: ACT APDC** (ACT Admitted Patient Data Collection)
- **Emergency Department: ACT EDDC** (ACT Emergency Department Data Collection)
- **Core Administration: ACT PAS** (Patient Administration System)
- **Statutory Registries: ACTCR** (ACT Cancer Registry), **ACT Perinatal Data Collection**

Northern Territory (NT)

- **Admitted Inpatients: NT IPAD** (NT Inpatient Activity Dataset)
- **Emergency Department: NT EDIS / EDDC** (Emergency Department Information System / Data Collection)
- **Statutory Registries: NTCR** (Northern Territory Cancer Registry), **NT Perinatal Data Collection**

These datasets support:

- Policy development
- Funding allocation
- Public reporting
- Research
- System performance monitoring

AIHW (2024) emphasises that reporting accuracy strengthens national health intelligence.

Data Validation and Auditing

Data validation ensures that information is complete, logical, and compliant with standards.

Common Validation Checks

- Missing fields
- Invalid codes
- Logical inconsistencies
- Incorrect sequencing
- Out-of-range values
- DRG anomalies

Auditing

Audits identify:

- Coding errors
- Documentation gaps
- Funding risks
- Compliance issues

Auditing strengthens data integrity and supports continuous improvement.

Analytics and Health Intelligence

Analytics transforms raw data into meaningful insights.

Key Analytical Tools

- Power BI
- Tableau
- SQL
- Excel advanced functions
- Predictive modelling tools

Common HIM Analytics

- Length-of-stay trends
- Readmission rates
- DRG shifts
- Coding variance
- Documentation improvement metrics
- ABF performance indicators

Analytics supports clinical improvement, funding accuracy, and strategic decision-making.

Predictive Analytics and Machine Learning

Machine learning models can predict:

- Patient risk
- Resource needs
- Coding anomalies
- Documentation gaps
- Funding impacts

AI-driven analytics strengthens organisational planning and supports proactive decision-making.

The HIM Role in Funding Integrity

HIM professionals protect funding integrity by ensuring:

- Accurate documentation
- Correct coding
- Reliable DRG assignment
- Strong audit trails
- Compliance with standards
- Transparent reporting

Funding integrity is essential for hospital sustainability and public trust.

Pathways to Becoming a Clinical Coder

Clinical Coders enter the profession through a combination of formal training and practical experience. In Australia, common pathways include:

- **Certificate IV in Clinical Classification** former qualification that is no longer available (HIMAA)
- **Diploma or Advanced Diploma in Health Administration** with coding streams
- **Bachelor or Master of Health Information Management** (graduates qualify as both HIMs and Clinical Coders)
- **On-the-job training programs** offered by hospitals and health services
- **Short courses** in ICD-10-AM, ACHI, ACS, and casemix fundamentals

Clinical Coders may progress into roles such as:

- Senior Clinical Coder
- Coding Auditor
- Casemix Analyst
- Documentation Improvement Specialist
- Coding Educator
- HIM Manager (with further tertiary study)

Salary Expectations for Data, Coding, and Funding Roles Australia (2024–2026)

Sources: Seek, Indeed, Labour Market Insights.

- Clinical Coder: AUD $65,000–$85,000
- Senior Clinical Coder: AUD $85,000–$110,000

- Coding Auditor/Educator: AUD $100,000–$125,000
- ABF Analyst: AUD $95,000–$130,000
- Health Data Scientist: AUD $110,000–$150,000

United States (AHIMA, 2024)

- Clinical Data Analyst: USD $75,000–$105,000
- Coding Auditor: USD $80,000–$115,000

United Kingdom (NHS, 2024)

- Information Analyst: £32,000–£42,000
- Senior Data Manager: £45,000–£55,000

Learning Framework: Strengthening Data and Funding Capability

- Build strong documentation and coding knowledge
- Learn analytics tools (Power BI, SQL, Tableau)
- Understand ABF and casemix principles
- Strengthen audit and validation skills
- Engage with AIHW, IHACPA, HIMAA resources
- Participate in data quality improvement projects
- Pursue advanced analytics training

Conclusion

Data quality, clinical coding, and funding integrity are central to the HIM profession. Accurate documentation, coding, reporting, and analytics support safe care, fair funding, and transparent governance. By strengthening data literacy, coding expertise, and analytical capability, HIM professionals play a vital role in shaping high-performing, sustainable healthcare systems.

Chapter 4: Privacy, FOI, and Ethical Information Release

Privacy, confidentiality, and ethical information release are central pillars of Health Information Management (HIM). As healthcare becomes increasingly digital, the risks associated with information misuse, breaches, and inappropriate disclosure grow significantly. HIM professionals must navigate complex legislation, high-stakes FOI requests, ethical dilemmas, and organisational pressures while upholding fairness, transparency, and integrity.

This chapter explores privacy obligations, FOI processes, ethical decision-making, governance frameworks, and the role of HIM professionals in protecting information integrity.

Privacy as a Foundation of HIM Practice

Privacy is a fundamental human right and a core HIM responsibility. Healthcare organisations must comply with strict privacy legislation to protect patient information and maintain public trust.

Key Privacy Legislation

- *Privacy Act 1988*
- Australian Privacy Principles (APPs)
- *Health Records Act 2001* (Vic)
- *Health Records and Information Privacy Act 2002* (NSW)
- GDPR (Europe)
- HIPAA (United States)

The Office of the Australian Information Commissioner (OAIC, 2024) emphasises that privacy compliance is essential for ethical and lawful information management.

Core Privacy Obligations

- Collect only necessary information

- Use information for legitimate purposes
- Secure data against breaches
- Provide individuals access to their own information
- Maintain transparency about information handling
- Ensure staff follow privacy policies and training

Privacy breaches can result in legal penalties, reputational damage, and harm to patients.

Confidentiality and Ethical Information Handling

Confidentiality requires HIM professionals to protect patient information from unauthorised access or disclosure.

Ethical Responsibilities

- Respect patient autonomy
- Protect sensitive information
- Avoid unnecessary sharing
- Apply legislation consistently
- Document decisions transparently
- Escalate concerns when needed

Ethical confidentiality extends beyond legal compliance, it reflects professional integrity and respect for human dignity.

Freedom of Information (FOI) in Healthcare

FOI legislation promotes transparency and accountability by allowing individuals to request access to documents held by public agencies.

Purpose of FOI

- Strengthen public trust
- Promote transparency
- Support accountability

- Enable individuals to access information about themselves or public decisions

FOI Workflow

FOI decision-making involves:

- Receiving and validating requests
- Locating relevant documents
- Reviewing content for sensitive information
- Assessing exemptions
- Consulting with stakeholders
- Applying the public interest test
- Issuing written decisions
- Releasing documents or refusing access

OVIC (2021) emphasises that FOI decisions must be fair, impartial, and well-reasoned.

Common FOI Exemptions

FOI legislation includes exemptions to protect sensitive information.

Key Exemptions

- **Personal privacy** — protects third-party personal information
- **Legal professional privilege** — protects confidential legal advice
- **Health and safety risks** — prevents harm to individuals
- **Law enforcement** — protects investigations and security
- **Cabinet documents** — protects government deliberations
- **Confidential commercial information** — protects business interests

HIM professionals must apply exemptions carefully and consistently.

Ethical Decision-Making in FOI and Privacy

Ethical decision-making is essential when handling sensitive information, especially in high-profile or complex FOI requests.

Ethical Principles

- **Integrity** — act honestly and transparently
- **Fairness** — apply legislation consistently
- **Respect** — consider the rights of all parties
- **Accountability** — document reasoning clearly
- **Courage** — make difficult decisions under pressure

Common Ethical Challenges

- Balancing privacy with transparency
- Managing high-profile or politically sensitive requests
- Handling requests involving vulnerable individuals
- Navigating organisational pressure
- Ensuring fairness in public interest assessments

Ethical HIM practice requires strong judgment, legislative knowledge, and professional courage.

Information Governance and Compliance

Information governance ensures that health information is managed ethically, securely, and in compliance with legislation.

Key Governance Components

- Privacy compliance
- FOI obligations
- Records management
- Cybersecurity
- Risk management
- Policy development
- Staff training

- Audit and monitoring

The Australian Digital Health Agency (ADHA, 2024) emphasises that governance is essential for safe digital health environments.

Records Management

Governed by:

- *Public Records Act 1973* (Vic)
- State archival authorities
- National digital health standards

Records must be accurate, complete, secure, retained appropriately, and disposed of lawfully.

High-Risk and High-Profile Information Release

Some FOI and privacy matters involve significant risk.

Examples of High-Risk Scenarios

- Requests involving public figures
- Sensitive mental health information
- Domestic violence or child protection cases
- Legal disputes
- Media-driven requests
- Requests involving multiple agencies

Risk Mitigation Strategies

- Consult legal teams
- Document reasoning thoroughly
- Apply exemptions consistently
- Conduct public interest tests carefully
- Escalate complex matters to senior governance leaders

High-risk information release requires advanced HIM expertise.

Global Perspectives on Privacy and Transparency

Privacy and transparency expectations vary globally, but common themes include:

- Stronger consumer rights
- Increased digital privacy regulation
- Expansion of global privacy frameworks
- Growth of digital identity systems
- International data sharing challenges
- Ethical AI governance

WHO (2023) emphasises that global digital health maturity requires robust privacy and governance frameworks.

Qualifications for FOI and Privacy Professionals

FOI Officers and Privacy Officers often come from diverse backgrounds. Common qualifications include:

- **Certificate IV or Diploma in Government (Information Management)**
- **Bachelor's degrees** in HIM, law, public administration, or information management
- **Specialised FOI training** from OVIC or OAIC
- **Privacy and data protection certifications**, such as:
    - IAPP CIPP/E (Certified Information Privacy Professional/Europe)
    - IAPP CIPM (Certified Information Privacy Manager)
    - OAIC (Office of the Australian Information Commissioner) Privacy Foundations courses

HIMs frequently oversee FOI and privacy teams due to their expertise in legislation, information governance, and ethical decision-making.

Salary Expectations for Privacy, FOI, and Governance Roles
Australia (2024–2026)
Sources: Seek, Indeed, Labour Market Insights.

- FOI/Privacy Officer: AUD $80,000–$105,000
- Senior Privacy Advisor: AUD $110,000–$135,000
- Information Governance Manager: AUD $120,000–$150,000
- Director of Governance / Chief Privacy Officer: AUD $150,000–$200,000

United States (IAPP & AHIMA, 2024)

- Privacy Analyst: USD $70,000–$95,000
- Compliance Manager: USD $100,000–$140,000
- Chief Privacy Officer: USD $150,000–$200,000

United Kingdom (NHS, 2024)

- Information Governance Officer: £32,000–£42,000
- FOI Manager: £38,000–£50,000
- Head of Information Governance: £50,000–£65,000

Learning Framework: Strengthening Privacy and FOI Capability

- Study privacy and FOI legislation
- Practice ethical decision-making
- Strengthen documentation and reasoning skills
- Engage in governance and compliance training
- Participate in FOI and privacy audits
- Pursue IAPP privacy certifications
- Build confidence in high-risk decision-making
- Engage with OVIC, OAIC, HIMAA resources

Conclusion

Privacy, FOI, and ethical information release are central to HIM practice. HIM professionals must balance transparency with confidentiality, apply legislation consistently, and uphold ethical standards in all decisions. By strengthening governance capability and ethical judgment, HIM professionals protect patient rights, support organisational integrity, and contribute to safe, trustworthy healthcare systems.

Chapter 5: Leadership, Stakeholder Management, and Workforce Development

Leadership is an essential capability for Health Information Management (HIM) professionals. As healthcare systems become more complex, digital, and regulated, HIM leaders must navigate organisational dynamics, influence stakeholders, build high-performing teams, and uphold ethical governance. Effective leadership strengthens data quality, privacy compliance, digital transformation, and workforce resilience.

This chapter explores leadership principles, communication strategies, stakeholder engagement, psychological safety, workforce capability uplift, and the development of professional identity within HIM.

Leadership in Health Information Management

HIM leadership extends beyond managing information, it involves guiding people, shaping culture, and influencing organisational strategy. HIM leaders must balance technical expertise with emotional intelligence, ethical judgment, and strategic thinking.

Core Leadership Responsibilities

- Supporting digital health transformation
- Ensuring privacy, FOI, and governance compliance
- Leading documentation and coding improvement
- Managing workforce capability and performance
- Building relationships with clinicians, executives, and IT teams
- Navigating organisational change
- Upholding ethical standards

Leadership is essential for advancing HIM practice and strengthening healthcare systems.

Communication as a Leadership Tool

Communication is one of the most powerful tools available to HIM leaders. Clear, respectful, and strategic communication supports collaboration, reduces conflict, and enhances organisational trust.

Key Communication Skills

- Active listening
- Clear articulation of complex information
- Tailoring messages to different audiences
- Providing constructive feedback
- Managing difficult conversations
- Communicating decisions transparently

Goleman (2021) emphasises that emotionally intelligent communication strengthens influence and teamwork.

Communicating with Clinicians

Clinicians respond best to communication that is:

- Evidence-based
- Respectful
- Focused on patient safety
- Practical and time-efficient

Communicating with Executives

Executives require:

- High-level summaries
- Risk assessments
- Funding implications
- Strategic recommendations

Effective communication builds credibility and trust.

Stakeholder Engagement and Relationship Management

HIM professionals interact with a wide range of stakeholders, including:

- Clinicians
- Nurses
- Executives
- IT teams
- Legal Advisors
- Privacy Officers
- FOI Officers
- Data Analysts
- External agencies

Strong stakeholder engagement ensures collaboration, reduces resistance, and supports successful digital and governance initiatives.

Principles of Effective Stakeholder Engagement

- Build relationships early
- Understand stakeholder priorities
- Communicate clearly and consistently
- Demonstrate empathy and respect
- Provide evidence-based recommendations
- Follow through on commitments
- Manage conflict constructively

Stakeholder engagement is essential for HIM leadership success.

Psychological Safety and Team Culture

Psychological safety is the belief that team members can speak up, ask questions, and admit mistakes without fear of embarrassment or punishment.

Edmondson (2019) emphasises that psychologically safe teams:

- Innovate more
- Learn faster
- Perform better
- Maintain stronger compliance
- Communicate more openly

How HIM Leaders Build Psychological Safety

- Encourage questions
- Respond to mistakes with curiosity, not blame
- Model respectful communication
- Invite diverse perspectives
- Provide constructive feedback
- Celebrate learning and improvement

Psychological safety strengthens team resilience and supports high-quality information management.

Workforce Capability and Professional Development

HIM leaders are responsible for developing workforce capability across coding, privacy, FOI, digital health, and data quality.

Key Workforce Development Strategies

- Mentoring and coaching
- Cross-training across HIM functions
- Professional development planning
- Coding and documentation education
- Privacy and FOI training
- Digital health literacy programs

- Performance management
- Recruitment and retention strategies

Workforce capability uplift ensures organisational readiness for digital transformation and governance challenges.

Professional Identity in HIM

Professional identity refers to the values, behaviours, and competencies that define a profession. A strong HIM identity supports confidence, ethical practice, and leadership development.

Elements of Professional Identity

- Ethical responsibility
- Data stewardship
- Privacy and confidentiality
- Governance expertise
- Digital health literacy
- Leadership and advocacy
- Commitment to lifelong learning

HIMAA (2023) emphasises that professional identity strengthens workforce resilience and organisational influence.

Building Professional Identity

- Engage in professional associations (HIMAA, AHIMA, IFHIMA, HIMSS)
- Pursue certifications
- Participate in conferences and CPD
- Seek mentorship
- Contribute to policy development
- Lead improvement initiatives

Professional identity supports career progression and leadership readiness.

Organisational Influence and Strategic Leadership

HIM leaders influence organisational strategy through:

- Policy development
- Risk management
- Digital transformation leadership
- Governance frameworks
- Documentation improvement
- Coding optimisation
- Data quality initiatives
- Privacy and FOI compliance

Strategic leadership strengthens organisational performance and supports safe, ethical healthcare.

Qualifications for Casemix and Funding Integrity Roles

Casemix Managers and ABF Analysts usually hold qualifications in:

- **Health Information Management**
- **Health Economics**
- **Statistics or Data Analytics**
- **Public Health**
- **Business or Finance (with healthcare experience)**

Additional training includes:

- IHACPA ABF education modules
- Coding audit certifications
- Data quality and reporting courses
- Statistical analysis training (R, Python, Power BI)

HIMs frequently lead casemix teams due to their expertise in coding, documentation, and funding integrity.

Salary Expectations for Leadership and Stakeholder Roles

Australia (2024–2026)

Sources: Seek, Indeed, Labour Market Insights.

- Senior HIM Officer: AUD $95,000–$120,000
- Team Leader / Supervisor: AUD $100,000–$130,000
- HIM Manager: AUD $120,000–$150,000
- Information Governance Manager: AUD $120,000–$150,000
- Director of Health Information Services: AUD $160,000–$220,000

United States (AHIMA, 2024)

- HIM Manager: USD $80,000–$120,000
- Director of HIM: USD $120,000–$160,000
- Chief Health Information Officer: USD $180,000–$250,000

United Kingdom (NHS, 2024)

- Senior Information Manager: £45,000–£55,000
- Head of Information Governance: £50,000–£65,000
- Director of Digital Health: £75,000–£130,000

Learning Framework: Strengthening Leadership Capability

- Develop emotional intelligence
- Strengthen communication skills
- Build stakeholder engagement strategies
- Foster psychological safety
- Lead workforce capability uplift
- Engage in professional associations
- Pursue leadership training

- Practice ethical decision-making
- Contribute to organisational strategy

Conclusion

Leadership is essential for advancing HIM practice and strengthening healthcare systems. By developing communication skills, stakeholder engagement strategies, psychological safety, and professional identity, HIM professionals can influence organisational culture, support digital transformation, and uphold ethical governance. Strong leadership ensures that HIM remains a respected, strategic, and future-ready profession.

Chapter 6: Building and Future-Proofing HIM Career

The Health Information Management (HIM) profession is evolving rapidly due to digital transformation, global interoperability, artificial intelligence, automation, and increasing governance complexity. To thrive in this dynamic environment, HIM professionals must adopt long-term strategies that strengthen digital capability, governance expertise, ethical judgment, leadership skills, and global awareness.

This chapter provides a comprehensive roadmap for building a resilient, future-ready HIM career, exploring professional identity, global workforce trends, emerging roles, and practical strategies for long-term success.

Understanding the Future HIM Landscape

The future of HIM will be shaped by technological innovation, global data exchange, and increasing regulatory demands. IFHIMA (2022) predicts that HIM professionals will increasingly act as digital governance leaders, AI auditors, and global data stewards.

Key Drivers of Change

- AI-assisted coding and automation
- Global interoperability (HL7, FHIR, SNOMED CT, ICD-11)
- Cybersecurity governance
- Digital identity systems
- Cloud-based EMRs
- Predictive analytics and machine learning
- Consumer-driven digital health
- International workforce mobility

Understanding these trends is essential for career planning and professional growth.

Developing Digital Resilience

Digital resilience refers to the ability to adapt to new technologies, workflows, and digital health environments. It is now a core HIM competency.

Strengthening Digital Literacy

HIM professionals must understand:

- EMR/EHR functionality
- Interoperability standards
- AI-assisted coding tools
- Digital identity systems
- Cybersecurity basics

Digital literacy supports safe, efficient, and compliant digital health environments.

Participating in Digital Health Projects

Hands-on experience accelerates learning and builds confidence.

Learning Automation Tools

Automation strengthens efficiency and reduces manual workload.

Examples include:

- Robotic Process Automation (RPA)
- Automated FOI redaction tools
- AI-driven data validation

Digital resilience ensures long-term employability and leadership potential.

Strengthening Governance and Ethical Capability

Governance is central to HIM practice and will become even more important as digital health expands.

Mastering Legislation

HIM professionals must understand:

- Privacy Act 1988
- FOI Act 1982
- Health Records Act 2001
- Public Records Act 1973
- GDPR – General Data Protection Regulation (European Union regulation)
- HIPAA – Health Insurance Portability and Accountability Act (United States federal law)

Practicing Ethical Decision-Making

Ethical HIM practice requires:

- Fairness
- Transparency
- Accountability
- Respect
- Courage

Leading Privacy and FOI Initiatives

OVIC (2021) emphasises that FOI decision-making requires strong reasoning and documentation.

Governance capability strengthens professional credibility and organisational influence.

Developing Advanced Analytical Skills

Analytics is essential for ABF, reporting, digital health, and strategic decision-making.

Learning Analytical Tools

- Power BI
- Tableau
- SQL
- Excel advanced functions
- Predictive modelling tools

Practicing Trend Analysis

Identify patterns in:

- Coding
- Documentation
- DRG shifts
- Length-of-stay trends
- Readmission rates

Strengthening Critical Thinking

Evaluate risks, interpret legislation, and make evidence-based decisions.

AIHW (2024) emphasises that advanced analytics supports policy development and funding integrity.

Building Leadership Capability

Leadership is essential for career progression and organisational influence.

Practicing Emotional Intelligence

Goleman (2021) highlights that emotional intelligence improves teamwork, conflict resolution, and influence.

Strengthening Communication Skills

Effective communication supports collaboration with:

- Clinicians
- Executives
- IT teams
- Legal advisors
- Privacy and FOI officers

Leading Through Digital Transformation

HIM leaders must guide teams through:

- System upgrades
- Workflow redesign
- Documentation improvement
- Governance changes

Fostering Psychological Safety

Edmondson (2019) emphasises that psychologically safe teams innovate more and perform better.

Leadership capability is essential for senior and executive HIM roles.

Building Global Competence

Global competence strengthens professional mobility and international career opportunities.

Studying International Standards

- ICD-11
- SNOMED CT
- GDPR
- HIPAA

Understanding Global Workforce Trends

IFHIMA (2022) notes that HIM roles are expanding globally due to digital health adoption.

Participating in Global Networks

Engage with:

- IFHIMA: International Federation of Health Information Management Associations
- AHIMA: American Health Information Management Association
- HIMSS: Healthcare Information and Management Systems Society

- IAPP: International Association of Privacy Professionals

Pursuing International Certifications

- AHIMA RHIA/RHIT
- IAPP privacy certifications
- HIMSS digital health certifications

Global competence enhances career resilience and mobility.

Emerging HIM Roles of the Future

Digital transformation is creating new HIM roles worldwide.

Emerging Roles

- AI Auditor
- Digital Health Strategist
- Interoperability Specialist
- Cybersecurity Compliance Officer
- Global Health Data Analyst
- Digital Identity Manager
- Chief Health Information Officer (CHIO)
- Chief Data Officer (CDO)

These roles require advanced digital literacy, governance expertise, and leadership capability.

Building a Strategic Professional Portfolio

A professional portfolio demonstrates capability, leadership, and readiness for advanced roles.

Key Portfolio Components

- Professional achievements
- Coding audits
- FOI decisions
- Privacy assessments

- Digital health projects
- Data quality improvements
- Leadership examples
- Governance contributions
- Certifications and Continuing Professional Development activities

A strong portfolio supports promotions, leadership roles, and global opportunities.

Salary Expectations for Future-Ready HIM Professionals

Australia (2024–2026)

Sources: Seek, Indeed, Labour Market Insights.

- Early-Career Roles: AUD $70,000–$85,000
- Mid-Career Roles: AUD $95,000–$130,000
- Senior Roles: AUD $120,000–$160,000
- Executive Roles: AUD $160,000–$300,000

United States (AHIMA & HIMSS, 2024)

- HIM Manager: USD $80,000–$120,000
- Director of HIM: USD $120,000–$160,000
- CHIO/CDO: USD $180,000–$250,000

United Kingdom (NHS, 2024)

- HIM Manager: £45,000–£60,000
- Head of Information Governance: £50,000–£65,000
- Director of Digital Health: £75,000–£130,000

Global (IFHIMA, 2023)

Salary ranges increase with digital maturity, governance complexity, and organisational size.

Learning Framework: Future-Proofing Your HIM Career

- Strengthen digital literacy
- Master governance and legislation
- Develop analytical capability
- Build leadership skills
- Engage in professional associations
- Pursue certifications
- Adopt a global perspective
- Create a professional portfolio
- Commit to lifelong learning

Recommended Professional Development Pathways

To advance in HIM careers, professionals often pursue:

- **Postgraduate degrees** (Master of HIM, Master of Health Informatics, Master of Data Science)
- **Leadership qualifications** (Graduate Certificate in Leadership, MBA)
- **Privacy and FOI certifications**
- **Digital health and interoperability training**
- **Coding audit and CDI certifications**
- **Professional memberships** (HIMAA, IFHIMA, IAPP, HIMSS)

These pathways strengthen leadership capability, digital literacy, and governance expertise.

Conclusion

Future-proofing your HIM career requires strategic planning, continuous learning, and adaptability. By strengthening digital, governance, analytical, and leadership capabilities, HIM professionals can lead the future of healthcare and shape high-performing, ethical, and digitally mature health systems. The future of HIM is bright, and belongs to professionals who embrace innovation, integrity, and lifelong growth.

APPENDICES

This section consolidates all appendices into a single, structured reference resource for HIM professionals, Clinical Coders, Privacy Officers, FOI Practitioners, Digital Health Specialists, and Healthcare Leaders.

Appendix A: FOI Decision-Making Template

Purpose: To support consistent, transparent, and defensible FOI decision-making aligned with OVIC and legislative requirements.

FOI Assessment Template:

- Applicant details
- Request description
- Scope clarification
- Document search summary
- Exemptions considered
- Public interest test
- Third-party consultation
- Decision rationale
- Release schedule
- Review rights
- Record of communications

Appendix B: Privacy Breach Response Flowchart

1. Identify the Breach Unintended disclosure, loss, or unauthorised access.

2. Contain the Breach Secure systems, revoke access, isolate affected data.

3. Assess the Risk Evaluate sensitivity, individuals affected, potential harm.

4. Notify Affected Individuals Provide clear, timely communication.

5. Notify OAIC (if required) Mandatory under the Notifiable Data Breaches Scheme.

6. Implement Corrective Actions Training, policy updates, system changes.

7. Document the Incident Maintain a complete audit trail.

Appendix C: Coding Audit Checklist

Documentation Review:

- Completeness
- Specificity
- Alignment with clinical intent

Coding Review:

- ICD-10-AM accuracy
- ACHI procedure coding
- ACS compliance
- Sequencing correctness
- DRG validation
- Comorbidity capture
- Funding impact analysis

Audit Outcomes:

- Error rate
- DRG shifts
- Education needs
- CDI opportunities

Appendix D: Digital Health Maturity Assessment

Assessment Domains:

- EMR/EHR optimisation

- Interoperability readiness (HL7, FHIR, SNOMED CT, ICD11)
- Cybersecurity controls
- Workforce digital literacy
- Governance frameworks
- Analytics capability
- Automation and AI adoption

Maturity Levels:

- Emerging
- Developing
- Established
- Advanced
- Transformational

Appendix E: Professional Portfolio Guide
Portfolio Components:

- Key achievements
- Coding audits and outcomes
- FOI decisions
- Privacy assessments
- Digital health projects
- Governance contributions
- Leadership examples
- Certifications and Continuing Professional Development
- Research or publications

Purpose: Supports promotions, leadership roles, and global career mobility.

Appendix F: Clinical Coding & Casemix Management
Introduction

Clinical coding and casemix management are central to hospital funding, performance monitoring, and national reporting. HIM professionals and Clinical Coders manage millions of dollars in casemix-based revenue, making accuracy essential.

Role of Clinical Coders

Clinical Coders translate clinical documentation into:

- ICD-10-AM diagnosis codes
- ACHI procedure codes
- ACS sequencing rules
- DRG classifications

Their work directly influences:

- ABF funding
- Clinical benchmarking
- National reporting
- Research and epidemiology
- Organisational compliance

Casemix and Funding Integrity

Casemix determines:

- Funding allocation
- Resource utilisation
- Benchmarking
- Strategic planning

Under ABF:

- DRGs → NWAUs → Dollar value
- Incorrect coding → Under-funding or over-funding
- Funding discrepancies → Thousands or millions of dollars

HIM professionals act as **financial stewards.**

High-Impact Coding Errors

Examples:

- Missing acute renal failure → DRG downgrade
- Incorrect sepsis coding → Loss of complexity weighting
- Failure to code major procedures → Significant under-funding
- Incorrect sequencing → DRG shift
- Missing comorbidities → Reduced NWAU

Coding Audits and Quality Assurance

Audit types:

- Internal
- External (IHACPA, state departments)
- Targeted
- Concurrent

Audit focus:

- Documentation completeness
- Diagnosis specificity
- Procedure accuracy
- ACS compliance
- DRG validation
- Funding impact

HIM Leadership in Casemix

HIM leaders:

- Oversee coding teams
- Manage audits
- Educate clinicians

- Collaborate with finance
- Monitor DRG shifts
- Lead CDI initiatives
- Ensure IHACPA compliance

Casemix leadership requires advanced analytical and governance capability.

Appendix G: Clinical Documentation Improvement (CDI)

Introduction

CDI enhances documentation accuracy, specificity, and completeness. It strengthens coding quality, ABF integrity, clinical communication, and medico-legal protection.

Purpose of CDI

CDI ensures documentation:

- Reflects true clinical care
- Supports accurate coding
- Captures comorbidities and complications
- Aligns with ACS requirements
- Supports DRG accuracy
- Enhances patient safety

Key CDI Activities

Documentation Review

Review of:

- Progress notes
- Discharge summaries
- Operative reports
- Diagnostic results
- Medication charts

Clarification Queries

Issued when documentation is:

- Ambiguous
- Incomplete
- Inconsistent
- Missing key details

Queries must be clear, respectful, non-leading, and evidence-based.

Clinician Education

Topics include:

- Documentation specificity
- Comorbidity capture
- Funding impact
- ACS requirements
- DRG implications

CDI and Funding Integrity

CDI strengthens ABF accuracy by ensuring:

- Correct DRG assignment
- Accurate NWAU calculation
- Complete comorbidity capture
- Reliable cost-weight application
- Transparent audit trails

CDI Metrics

- Query response rates
- Documentation completeness
- DRG shifts
- Comorbidity capture rates
- Length-of-stay alignment

- Audit outcomes

Conclusion

CDI is essential for coding accuracy, funding integrity, clinical communication, and organisational performance. HIM professionals lead CDI programs and strengthen documentation quality across the health system.

GLOSSARY OF TERMS

ABF (Activity-Based Funding)

A funding model used in Australia that allocates hospital funding based on the complexity and volume of patient care. ABF relies heavily on accurate clinical coding and casemix data.

ACHI (Australian Classification of Health Interventions)

The national classification system for coding procedures and interventions performed in Australian hospitals.

ACS (Australian Coding Standards)

Rules and guidelines that Clinical Coders must follow when assigning ICD-10-AM and ACHI codes.

AI (Artificial Intelligence)

Technology that uses algorithms and machine learning to perform tasks such as coding assistance, predictive analytics, automation, and anomaly detection.

AI-Assisted Coding

The use of artificial intelligence tools to support Clinical Coders by suggesting codes based on clinical documentation. Human validation remains essential.

Audit Log

A system-generated record of user activity, used to monitor access, detect breaches, and support cybersecurity governance.

Casemix

A method of categorising patient types based on diagnoses, procedures, complexity, and resource use. Casemix determines hospital funding under ABF.

CDI (Clinical Documentation Improvement)

A structured program aimed at improving the accuracy, specificity, and completeness of clinical documentation to support coding accuracy, patient safety, and funding integrity.

Clinical Coding

The process of translating clinical documentation into ICD-10-AM and ACHI codes for reporting, funding, research, and analytics.

Clinical Documentation

Written or electronic records created by clinicians that describe patient care, diagnoses, procedures, and clinical decision-making.

Comorbidity

A condition that exists alongside the principal diagnosis and may impact patient complexity, treatment, and funding.

Confidentiality

The ethical and legal obligation to protect patient information from unauthorised access or disclosure.

Data Quality

The accuracy, completeness, consistency, validity, and reliability of health information.

Digital Health

The use of digital technologies such as EMRs, telehealth, AI, and interoperability standards to improve healthcare delivery.

Digital Identity

A secure digital credential used to verify a person's identity in digital health systems.

DRG (Diagnosis Related Group)

A classification system that groups patient episodes based on diagnoses, procedures, and complexity. DRGs determine ABF funding.

EHR (Electronic Health Record)

A digital record of a patient's health information that can be shared across multiple healthcare organisations.

EMR (Electronic Medical Record)

A digital version of a patient's medical chart within a single healthcare organisation.

Encryption

A cybersecurity method that protects data by converting it into unreadable code unless accessed with authorised credentials.

FHIR (Fast Healthcare Interoperability Resources)

A modern interoperability standard that enables real-time data exchange between digital health systems.

FOI (Freedom of Information)

Legislation that allows individuals to request access to documents held by public agencies, promoting transparency and accountability.

GDPR (General Data Protection Regulation)

European privacy legislation governing the collection, use, and protection of personal data.

Governance

Frameworks and processes that ensure information is managed ethically, securely, and in compliance with legislation.

Health Information Management (HIM)

A profession focused on managing health information across privacy, coding, digital health, governance, analytics, and funding.

HIPAA (Health Insurance Portability and Accountability Act)

US legislation governing health information privacy and security.

HL7 (Health Level Seven)

A messaging standard used for exchanging clinical and administrative data between systems.

ICD-10-AM (International Classification of Diseases, 10th Revision, Australian Modification)

The classification system used in Australia for coding diagnoses.

ICD-11

The latest global classification system for diseases, developed by the World Health Organization.

IHACPA (Independent Hospital and Aged Care Pricing Authority)

The Australian authority responsible for setting ABF pricing, NWAU values, and cost weights.

Interoperability

The ability of digital systems to exchange, interpret, and use information seamlessly.

Length of Stay (LOS)

The number of days a patient spends in hospital. LOS influences DRG assignment and funding.

LOINC (Logical Observation Identifiers Names and Codes)

A global standard for coding laboratory and clinical observations.

Machine Learning

A type of AI that identifies patterns in data and makes predictions or decisions.

Medico-Legal Documentation

Clinical documentation that may be used in legal proceedings or investigations.

NWAU (National Weighted Activity Unit)

The unit used to measure hospital activity under ABF. Each DRG has a specific NWAU value.

Over-Coding

Assigning codes that exaggerate patient complexity or do not align with documentation. Over-coding is a compliance risk.

Predictive Analytics

The use of statistical models and machine learning to predict future outcomes such as patient risk or resource needs.

Principal Diagnosis

The condition chiefly responsible for the patient's admission to hospital.

Privacy

The right of individuals to control how their personal information is collected, used, and disclosed.

Procedure Coding

Assigning ACHI codes to surgical or non-surgical interventions.

Public Interest Test

An FOI requirement that weighs the benefits of disclosure against potential harm.

Ransomware

Malicious software that encrypts data and demands payment for its release.

Records Management

The systematic control of records throughout their lifecycle, including creation, storage, access, and disposal.

Risk of Mortality (ROM)

A measure of the likelihood that a patient may die during an episode of care. ROM influences DRG complexity.

Sequelae

Conditions that arise as a direct result of a previous disease or injury.

SNOMED CT

A global clinical terminology used for interoperability and structured clinical documentation.

Stakeholder Engagement

The process of collaborating with clinicians, executives, IT teams, and other stakeholders to achieve HIM objectives.

Telehealth

The delivery of healthcare services using digital communication technologies.

Under-Coding

Failing to capture all relevant diagnoses or procedures, resulting in reduced funding and inaccurate reporting.

VAED (Victorian Admitted Episodes Dataset)

A dataset containing information on admitted patient episodes in Victoria.

VEMD (Victorian Emergency Minimum Dataset)

A dataset containing information on emergency department presentations in Victoria.

Workflow Optimisation

Improving processes to increase efficiency, accuracy, and staff satisfaction.

BIBLIOGRAPHY

Australian Digital Health Agency. (2024). *National digital health strategy.*

Australian Government Labour Market Insights. (2024). *Health information management salary data.*

Australian Institute of Health and Welfare. (2024). *Hospital data quality and auditing framework.*

Edmondson, A. (2019). *The fearless organization: Creating psychological safety in the workplace.* Wiley.

Goleman, D. (2021). *Emotional intelligence: Why it can matter more than IQ.* Bantam Books.

Health Information Management Association of Australia. (2023). *HIM competencies framework.*

HIMSS. (2024). *Digital health workforce report.*

Independent Hospital and Aged Care Pricing Authority. (2022). *Activity based funding model overview.*

International Federation of Health Information Management Associations. (2022). *Global HIM workforce report.*

NHS Digital. (2024). *Information management and digital health salary bands.*

Office of the Australian Information Commissioner. (2024). *Privacy Act 1988 guidelines.*

Office of the Victorian Information Commissioner. (2021). *Freedom of Information guidelines.*

World Health Organization. (2023). *Digital health and data governance framework.*